RESETTING MENOPAUSE:
Eliminate Symptoms And Feel Young Again

By

I0696351

LINDA A. ROBERTS

Table Of Content

Introduction

Menopause is a subject that many people have misunderstood for a long time. The majority of people, including males, frequently believed that menopause was an illness. In the past, people believed that menopausal women were depressed and that their time was running out. Others believed that menopausal women were simply weary of having sex. However, in the present period, opinions toward menopause have significantly improved.

These days, going through menopause is common. Thankfully, a wealth of knowledge is also readily available online, making this stage of life manageable and easy to navigate. It's widely acknowledged that while some people find the menopause transition to be pleasant, others find it to be intimidating due to the ease with which information can be accessed. The best part is that talking about menopause has allowed women who find it difficult to cope to get the help they most need.

It's possible that you chose this guide because menopause is causing you anxiety. Menopause is not admirable at all, in actuality. Even with the wealth of knowledge that can be found online, in periodicals, and in newspapers, millions of women still experience anxiety when considering menopause or going through it later in life. Every other day, new and unfounded worries surface, causing mental and emotional distress in women. In actuality, some of the information provided to media outlets frequently contradicts medical advice. It's possible that the false impressions you pick up from the things you read, watch, and listen to have affected you. Women frequently become so terribly anxious that they quit taking their prescriptions.

While you read this book, you'll be looking for reliable and valuable information. You may be searching for all-encompassing information to improve your health both during and after menopause reversal. Most likely, menopausal symptoms have begun to interfere with your day-to-day activities. It's also possible that you haven't had any symptoms, but you've been feeling uneasy about your general health lately. You may have begun making certain adjustments to enhance your overall health and well-being. Regrettably, changes in health can cause a variety of frustrations. You could have dedicated hours to your regular gym visits. You stay away from unhealthy foods and stick to salads, grilled chicken, and fish. But the weight scale's numbers never seem to move. Even worse, even with your daily exercise regimen, you may find that you are gaining weight rather than reducing it.

Menopause is now an average period that women go through, as was previously said. Unexpectedly, we frequently ponder how our grandmothers got through this stage without prescription drugs and diagnostic procedures. Maybe they adopted healthier habits, or maybe they were fortunate enough to avoid becoming addicted to junk food or sweets. We can all agree that women in this generation will struggle with post-menopause for more than a third of their lives, regardless of their personal reasons. We, therefore, have a responsibility to try our best to understand the potential consequences both during and after menopause.

To be clear, you should not conclude from reading this book that you can get by without professional medical assistance. It would be best if you didn't rely solely on the information in this book to achieve your ideal reset metabolism health for menopause. Consequently, I recommend that you speak with your physician, who specializes in the treatment of women. Following medical guidance will ensure that you maintain good health and are productive for as long as feasible, in addition to ensuring that you take good care of yourself during and following menopause. Becoming best friends with this guide is the ideal way to begin your journey towards bettering your well-being. It would help if you then remembered to make an appointment with your physician or other medical specialist.

I have compiled the most current and helpful material that has been scientifically shown to assist menopausal ladies from my vast research on gynecology and menopausal women. I will thus walk you through the most critical lifestyle and health decisions in this guide so that you can live a full, vibrant, and joyful life.

I honestly can't wait to guide you down the correct route and help you triumph over the challenges of controlling and managing menopause. This manual is organized into several chapters, each of which covers a typical problem that menopausal women encounter on a regular basis. First, you will discover the facts of menopause and acquire a deeper understanding of many health concerns, such as hot flashes, sleep, sex, moods, emotions, food, and exercise, among other things. I urge you to read this guide through from start to finish, even if you are only interested in reading about specific menopausal issues. There are many valuable suggestions on how to enhance your health and well-being in every chapter.

Remember that there are many benefits to receiving preventative treatment, especially if you are over 40. Frequently, the medical conditions linked to aging are the result of poor lifestyle choices. After going through what you are, you have to realize that changing your lifestyle is something you can do at any time. More significantly, we must acknowledge that, as we age over 40, our health can change in unanticipated ways. We are unsure of the next issue that may arise in comparison to our 205. It was

reasonable to presume that you were physically fit, well, and in good health back then; this isn't the case as you become older. Even though you may feel OK, in real life, you are coping with a condition that is becoming worse every other day. This implies that you cannot ignore your health and remain indifferent. The good news is that you made the proper decision to manage menopause and begin your journey towards improved health successfully.

You are going to experience notable changes in your health once you have finished reading and fully understanding the advice in this book. You'll discover how to feel alive once you regain your sense of well-being. You'll eat better, exercise more, and even have better interactions with your loved ones on a personal level. Yes, the menopause self-care strategy described in this book will help you monitor your health closely each day. How nice would it be to awaken to a peaceful, clear, and joyful inner state and to finally recognize that you have achieved sustainable weight loss at the beginning of the day? All the information you require to restore your health and lead a comfortable life during the turbulent menopausal years will be covered in this guide.

I'll start now!

Chapter 1

Whose Body Am I Living In?

Could we, for a second, get real?

The menopause is so tricky. It's not easy to deal with issues like insomnia, unstable moods, memory loss, hot flashes, thinning hair, dry vagina, and decreased libido. Managing menopause is not like managing a severe case of the flu that passes in a few weeks. Over the course of ten years, our bodies undergo significant changes. The symptoms don't seem to be related to anything. They appear and disappear without notice. Hormones that have kept you joyful, focused, invigorated, and burning fat are gone.

They are missed. However, they are leaving. We experience this hormonal drop alone, and there aren't many answers available to ease the turbulent, crazy, and wild ride. I wish to alter that.

Why don't women talk about their menopausal journeys more frequently? Why aren't we providing women with more effective lifestyle tools to address this? Why do ladies not assist one another during this process? It's an intense sport, menopause. A training manual on how to get ready for this expedition would be helpful. We must rely on one another and support one another.

I've spent the last ten years navigating the menopause, and I now understand that I wasn't alone. Far too many ladies are going through similar things. For some, it's even worse. When women reach this stage of life, they battle with their health. When your hormones start to drop, it can be really unpleasant. Countless individuals have contacted me. I find your stories to be moving to the extent that they motivated me to pen this book.

My health took a turn for the worse when I turned forty. I was in the best physical form of my life when I turned 40. I was pretty sure that getting older would be easy. But at the age of 42, my health had collapsed. My reality became hot flashes, sleeplessness, memory loss, mood swings, and unexpected weight gain. I had the impression that an extraterrestrial had taken over my body and that I was living in someone else's. My sense of control over my health had vanished. The most challenging aspect of this trip has been realizing that none of the old strategies I had for improving my health have worked.

The complicated and erratic nature of menopausal symptoms is one of the most challenging aspects of the transition. It's difficult to identify what starts them, and we frequently have no idea when or how long they will last. Many of us have learned to accept our PMS symptoms for years. That was nothing compared to the menopausal transition. Just before our periods, we experience a brief hormonal shift known as PMS. We've discovered strategies to deal with them, and lots of chocolate is one of those strategies. However, the hormonal path during menopause is distinct. Not everything is as predictable. Symptoms appear at the most inconvenient times and come and go without warning. This wild hormonal roller coaster is accompanied by a wide range of emotions. Our mood swings might be detrimental to our relationships. Anger and anger start to appear frequently. Some of us discover that we are shouting more at our partners and children. Even the tiniest events have the power to agitate us. The hardest thing is that we frequently don't understand why. Oftentimes, we feel agitated as we go about it.

Thousands of women whom I have guided through menopause have confided in me that they have lost all sense of joy in life. When the little things that used to make you happy as a child no longer excite you, it can be frustrating. For many women, these are the years when their memory deteriorates. Far too many people find themselves forgetting identities and scrambling to find words in the middle of a conversation. For many menopausal women, a good night's sleep can seem like a thing of the past. We are readily roused by any movement or sound.

Once we're awake, we try to fall back asleep by tossing and turning for hours. We have to get out of bed a lot to change our clothes and linens because we wake up so sweaty many nights. There were far too many of us at this time who would do anything to feel refreshed when we woke up.

Add to that weight gain. Let's briefly discuss weight gain. That's not just. Do you believe that despite eating the same or possibly less and exercising more, all you are managing to do is put on weight? Menopause can come as a surprise. We feel too young to be going through menopause far too often. Your mother had gone through menopause when she grew older.

Even though this path may be challenging for you, I want you to step back from your symptoms for a little while in order to see things from a different angle. Going through menopause is not necessary. That's right, it is. Your amazing body is requesting assistance, and that is why you are experiencing these symptoms. It's not necessary for you to fight through them. You own far greater power than that. The menopause journey offers an exquisite chance to become in tune with your body and discover its requirements.

Each person has various needs. My goal is to assist you in creating a lifestyle tailored to your body's needs.

Ailments are gifts. Although symptoms don't feel that way when they're happening, your body would communicate with you through them if it had a language. Avoid painting the process as a villain. Listen to it and tune in. There is a reason why these symptoms appear. I understand the difficulty of residing in a body that does not feel like your own. I am aware that these symptoms could make you feel miserable. You feel like you've tried everything to feel better, but nothing seems to be helping. You have tried a plethora of herbs, vitamins, medications, therapies, and diets in an effort to feel normal once more. You are entirely frustrated and at a loss for words. You're with me. Aid is en route. Consider this book to be a guide on how to make the menopausal transition easier. The menopause might be an inside-out experience for you.

I want to show you how to live a lifestyle that recognizes the wisdom your body has within, one that supports the changes occurring inside of you rather than searching for something external to treat your symptoms. Your external experience will alter as a result. I want to provide you with the knowledge and skills to work with, rather than against, your body by teaching you the language that it speaks.

You'll see that my passion is science. Knowing something works isn't sufficient for me; I also want to know why it works. My whole approach to healing has been based on the use of techniques that are not only shown to be successful but also supported by scientific evidence. One of the most shocking things I learned during my menopausal journey was that postmenopausal women are more likely to suffer from diseases, including breast cancer, ovarian cancer, heart disease, diabetes, dementia, and Alzheimer's. I was curious as to why it was the situation. What occurs that predisposes women to so many illnesses? I found that hormones function similarly to a symphony. Every instrument contributes to the creation of a lovely piece of music. The entire piece will not sound right if one of the instruments breaks. Disease arises from this breakdown of a few hormones. Not only may hormone balancing help us maintain our sanity during menopause, but it can also save our lives.

My goal is to make this clear to women. We can assist a woman in avoiding significant illnesses like cancer, heart disease, dementia, Alzheimer's, and even osteoporosis if we make course corrections during her menopausal years.

It is a privilege to accompany you on this journey. I firmly think that everything that occurs in our lives has a purpose. I am aware that my menopause difficulties occurred in order to provide support for thousands of ladies going through a similar situation.

When you read this book, keep an open mind. Although many of the lifestyle strategies I suggest are state-of-the-art, they can go against everything you have been taught thus far. Science teaches us in a distinct way. The world in which we currently reside is not the same as it was decades ago. We must approach menopause differently as a result.

For you, I have fantastic news. You have control over these symptoms no matter where you are in the menopausal journey. And swiftly. It can be as easy as adopting lifestyle adjustments that will accommodate the hormonal decrease you are going through; it doesn't require a miracle medication. I can't wait to share with you the lifestyle skills that have made this difficult journey more accessible for me and thousands of my patients. Miracle drugs would not exist. The human body is powerful. The female body has such a fantastic design. Our purpose in being created was to bear another human child. That's really cool. However, this design undergoes a significant change when we approach menopause. To treat that transition, you don't need an antidepressant drug or a miracle herb. To adapt your lifestyle to the changes occurring within you, a change is necessary.

Understanding is power. You will feel more in control of your body the more you comprehend what it is going through. Hormone knowledge is complicated. In order to help you work with, rather than against, your hormones, this book aims to simplify them for you. Your symptoms are curable. Menopause is a time when you can thrive. You've been taught that you are weaker than this. Returning that authority to you makes me very happy.

Chapter 2

You Are Not Losing Your Mind…You Are Loosing Hormones

It's possible that you've observed that you're finding it difficult to focus. You're having trouble finishing tasks at work or at home. You feel nervous and stressed, but you're not sure why because nothing seems to have changed on the outside.

You recognize someone you see, but you can't quite place them. Then, you discover that you can no longer remember some frequent phrases. You are losing your memory, and at this stage, you begin to feel a little anxious about whether you have a mental health problem or are suffering from a brain condition. Despite your best efforts, you are unable to overcome your mental fog. You have trouble remembering things that happened recently. You have depressive symptoms and a sense of being trapped in a world of gray.

Perhaps you even sit there in tears, unable to comprehend what's happening. You begin to worry that you're going to have a mental breakdown and that you're going insane. Most people are unaware that your hormones may have gone astray, which could be the root of all of that.

Many women experience unnecessary suffering as a result of failing to consider the possible physical symptoms in addition to the emotional ones. However, hormones can make you feel as though you're losing your mind. You might even question what's wrong with you and worry that you've somehow lost yourself all of a sudden.

Most people presume something serious when their hormones are out of balance, but there's no reason to panic. Testing your hormone levels should be your initial course of action. Each and every hormone has the power to influence both your brain and your mood. Individuals who have an imbalance in their thyroid hormones may suffer from sadness and memory loss.

Emotional and mental disorders are known to be brought on by imbalanced thyroid hormones. Occasionally, testosterone levels fluctuate, rising or falling short of average. Your mood may shift, and you may feel like a different person when that occurs. It may cause mental fog and difficulty focusing. Memory loss may occur if you have abnormalities in either progesterone or estrogen.

You may be really upset one minute and pleased the next, and you may cry at the drop of a hat. Your emotions suddenly become erratic because progesterone loses its ability to function as a mood stabilizer in the brain when it becomes out of balance.

Despite being the most common source of changes in the body, mind, and emotions, hormones are also the most ignored. The good news is that you'll feel normal again once things are balanced.

Chapter 3
Welcome To Menopause

What is menopause?

A woman enters menopause, a stage of life that ends when she no longer gets her periods. This stage, which is sometimes referred to as the "change of life," marks the end of a woman's ability to become pregnant. In fact, a lot of medical professionals refer to the phase of life when a woman's hormone levels start to fluctuate as menopause. After a year without a menstrual period, the menopause is considered complete.

Perimenopause is the term used to describe the transitional period preceding menopause. A woman's ovaries produce fewer mature eggs during this period of transition preceding menopause, and ovulation becomes erratic. Progesterone and estrogen production both decline at the same time. A decrease in the levels of estrogen is the primary cause of the majority of menopausal symptoms.

When does menopause occur?

Menopause can indeed occur at any age, although it typically occurs at 51. This includes the mid-50s and later. Those who smoke and are underweight typically go through menopause earlier than those who are overweight. A woman typically experiences menopause about the same age as her mother.

Menopause can occur for reasons other than those that are natural. These consist of:

- Premature menopause: When ovarian failure happens before the age of forty, premature menopause may result. It could be linked to ovarian blood supply-impairing surgery, radiation exposure, chemotherapy, or smoking. Primary ovarian insufficiency is another term for premature ovarian failure.

- Surgical menopause: After radiation of the pelvis, including the ovaries, in premenopausal women or after the removal of one or both ovaries, surgical menopause may ensue. The menopause ends abruptly as a result. Compared to women who would experience menopause naturally, they frequently experience more severe menopausal symptoms.

What are the symptoms of menopause?

The most typical signs of menopause are these. However, each woman may have a unique set of symptoms. While some people experience fewer, milder symptoms, others deal with more severe, frequent problems. Menopause symptoms and indicators could include:

1) Hot Flashes

Flush or hot flashes are by far the most typical menopausal symptoms. Approximately 75% of women experience these abrupt, fleeting, recurring temperature spikes. Hot flashes typically begin before a woman's previous menstruation. Hot flashes last two years or fewer for 80% of women. Fewer women than men have hot flashes for longer than two years. There appears to be a clear correlation between these flashes and declining estrogen levels. The frequency and intensity of hot flashes differ from woman to woman. A woman may experience an increase in heart rate in addition to a rise in skin temperature during a hot flash. The body attempts to lower its temperature as a result, which generates abrupt sweat. Additionally, dizziness and heart palpitations may accompany this symptom.

Night sweats are the term for hot flashes that occur during the night. It's possible for a lady to wake up perspiring and need to change out of her pajamas and bed linens.

2) Vaginal atrophy

The thinning and drying out of the urethral and vaginal tissues is known as vaginal atrophy. This can result in urinary tract infections, cystitis, vaginitis, and pain during intercourse.

3) Relaxation of the pelvic muscles

The danger of the uterus, bladder, urethra, or rectum bulging into the vagina increases when the pelvic muscles relax, which can result in urine incontinence.

4) Cardiac effects

Menopause symptoms can include irregular sensations, including numbness, prickling, tingling, increased sensitivity, cardiac palpitations, and fast heartbeat.

5) Hair growth

Some women may experience a loss of hair on their scalp or an increase in facial hair due to hormonal changes.

6) Mental health

Despite the widespread belief that menopause may have a detrimental impact on mental health, a number of studies have shown that menopausal women have no more levels of stress, anxiety, sadness, rage, or uneasiness than women of the same age who are still menstruating. Fatigue, irritability, insomnia, and anxiousness are psychological and emotional symptoms that can be linked to age, changing roles, and estrogen deficiency.

How do I stop having hot flashes?

A drop in estrogen levels causes hot flashes. Your body temperature fluctuates as a result of your glands releasing more hormones in reaction, which alters the thermostat in your brain. Many women have found that hormone therapy helps to reduce some of the discomfort associated with hot flashes. However, you and your healthcare practitioner should discuss your risk-against-benefit ratio before deciding to begin utilizing these hormones.

The Women's Health Initiative (WHI) of the National Institutes of Health teaches to learn more about women's health, particularly specifically hormone therapy. The hormone trial had two studies: the estrogen-alone study, which involved women without uteruses, and the estrogen-plus-progestin study, which involved women with uteruses. When it became clear that hormone therapy raised the risk of certain illnesses and did not help prevent heart disease, both trials came to an early conclusion. Women on estrogen-plus-progestin therapy had a higher risk of heart disease, according to follow-up studies. This risk was exceptionally high for women who began hormone therapy more than ten years after menopause.

The WHI advises women to adhere to FDA guidelines when it comes to hormone therapy (either estrogen-alone or estrogen-plus-progestin). It says that using hormone therapy to stop heart disease is not a good idea.

These products are authorized treatments for vulvar and vaginal atrophy symptoms, as well as mild to severe hot flashes. Hormone therapy should only be taken into consideration for women who are at a high risk of osteoporosis and are unable to use non-steroidal medications, even if it may be beneficial in preventing postmenopausal osteoporosis. The FDA advises using hormone therapy for the shortest amount of time and at the lowest doses possible in order to meet therapeutic objectives. Postmenopausal women who use hormone therapy or are thinking about starting should talk to their healthcare professionals about the potential advantages and disadvantages of the treatment.

Here are some doable recommendations for handling heat flashes:

- ✓ Wear layers of clothing so that you may take them off in the event of a heat flash.
- ✓ Steer clear of hot beverages and foods that can trigger hot flashes, such as alcohol, coffee, tea, and other hot drinks.
- ✓ When a hot flash begins, sip on a glass of cold water or fruit juice.
- ✓ Lessen your degree of stress. Anxiety can make hot flashes worse.
- ✓ Throughout the night, keep an ice pack or a thermos of ice water next to your bed.

- ✓ Wear clothing that lets your skin breathe and cotton sheets or undergarments.
- ✓ To identify potential triggers for your hot flashes, keep a journal or log of your symptoms.

Menopause treatment plans

Various treatments are available to assist or control menopausal symptoms, such as:

1) Hormonal therapy (HT)

During perimenopause and menopause, hormone treatment (HT) entails taking a combination of the female hormones progesterone and estrogen. The most typical way that HT is prescribed is as pills. On the other hand, vaginal lotions and skin patches can also be used to administer estrogen.

It would be best if you only decided to begin taking these hormones after discussing the advantages and disadvantages with your healthcare provider.

2) Estrogen therapy (ET)

Since the body can no longer produce estrogen on its own, estrogen therapy (ET) entails taking estrogen alone. Women who have had a hysterectomy are frequently administered ET. Prescription forms of estrogen include tablets, skin patches, and vaginal lotions.

It would help if you only decided to begin using this hormone after discussing the advantages and disadvantages with your healthcare provider.

3) Non-hormonal treatment

In order to reduce some of the menopausal symptoms, this kind of treatment frequently entails the use of other medications.

4) Estrogen alternatives

"Synthetic estrogens," or estrogen substitutes, such as ospemifene, alleviate vaginal atrophy symptoms without raising the risk of endometrial cancer.

5) Alternative therapies

Often referred to as bioidentical hormones, homeopathy and herbal remedies may provide some relief from specific menopause symptoms. Potency, safety, purity, and effectiveness are issues, though.

Chapter 4

Are There Any Links Between Alzheimer's Illness And Early Menopause?

- Early menopause may raise your risk of Alzheimer's disease, according to a recent study.
- The study suggests that hormone therapy may help reduce that risk.
- Despite its contentious history, professionals emphasize the value of hormone treatment in treating menopausal symptoms.

Women are twice as likely as males to get Alzheimer's disease and associated dementias, which affect 5.8 million individuals in the United States. According to a recent study, a woman's age during menopause may have an impact on her risk of developing Alzheimer's disease, but hormone therapy (HT) may be able to reduce that risk.

In order to search for evidence of beta-amyloid plaques and tau proteins, two indicators of Alzheimer's disease, researchers examined brain scans from 193 women and 99 men who did not have a diagnosis of the disease or any other type of dementia.

The researchers found that compared to men of the same age, women generally exhibited higher levels of amyloid plaques and tau accumulation in several brain regions. Progestin, a synthetic version of the progesterone hormone, is mixed with estrogen and was used by all the women in the study. According to the results, tau levels were higher in the brains of women who entered menopause before the age of forty, between the ages of forty and forty-five, or who began hormone therapy more than five years after the onset of menopause. However, the researchers also discovered that there was no increased risk for tau protein development in the brain in those who started using HT around the time they went through menopause, indicating that menopausal treatment may reduce the chance of Alzheimer's disease.

In the end, the researchers came to the conclusion that a woman's brain tau development may be influenced by entering menopause earlier in life and beginning hormone therapy later after menopause has started.

Although menopause strikes women on average at age 51, some may experience it earlier, usually before age 40. There is still debate on the history of hormone therapy and the connection between menopause and Alzheimer's disease. You undoubtedly have some questions after that. This is what we currently know.

Does dementia risk increase in women who go through early menopause?

Research has connected an earlier menopause to a higher chance of dementia in later life. Early menopause may be a significant sex-specific risk factor for the disease Alzheimer's, but more research is required. According to a study released last year, women who started menopause around age 45 were 30% more likely to be diagnosed with dementia before the age of 65 than women who started menopause at age 50.

Alzheimer's disease development is also believed to be influenced by additional risk factors.

- Genetics
- Heart disease
- High blood pressure
- Stroke
- Diabetes
- Obesity

Does estrogen deficiency cause Alzheimer's disease?

According to ACOG, a woman experiencing menopause experiences a decrease in the level of estrogen can lead to typical symptoms such as mood swings, hot flashes, and dry vagina. Having said that, while it hasn't been established beyond a reasonable doubt, some researchers have hypothesized that decreased estrogen levels may contribute to the onset of Alzheimer's. Long-term low estrogen levels have been shown to induce oxidative stress, which may have an effect on cognitive function.

We know that estrogen has a significant impact on the brain, that alterations can be observed in postmenopausal women, and that estrogen receptors are found in both gray and white matter. However, things "become a bit sticky" when discussing hormone therapy and Alzheimer's disease. Though this research did not surprise me, people are reluctant to advise, "Take hormone therapy to prevent Alzheimer's." This is not because it isn't true, but instead because it hasn't been demonstrated. We are aware of the significant effects that estrogen has on the brain. This could be proof that beginning hormone therapy treatment early can lower the chance of developing Alzheimer's disease in the future.

Chapter 5

Five Myths About Menopause That Should Be Dispelled Immediately

Even though talking about menopause is no longer completely taboo, not everyone feels comfortable doing so (particularly in the workplace, where many women spend so much of their time). As a result, falsehoods and misconceptions continue to exist. Here are some frequent but false misconceptions regarding this significant life stage that you should be aware of.

Myth 1: Hormone replacement therapy is dangerous

The truth is that HRT can safely relieve menopause symptoms like hot flashes, disrupted sleep, and vaginal/bladder issues for healthy women under 60 or younger than ten years post-menopause. In fact, an 18-year follow-up to the study that first sparked the public's fear of HRT revealed no increased risk of death from any cause for women who took HRT for five to seven years when compared to those who took a placebo. The original 2002 study indicated increased risks of breast cancer and heart disease, which garnered a lot of attention. However, the fact that the findings mainly pertained to older women on HRT was lost in the narrative. Dr. Ross continues, "The benefits of HRT generally outweigh the hazards when it comes to quality of life when it is used for the shortest feasible duration at the lowest effective dose." (HRT is not suggested for women with a history of blood clots, heart illness, liver disease, or certain cancers.)

Myth #2: Menopause symptoms don't last long

The fact is that menopause is a protracted process with up to ten years of symptoms. Fortunately, the majority of women experience a reduction in hot flashes, night sweats, and disturbed sleep as a result of their bodies adjusting to reduced amounts of progesterone and estrogen. Medication, especially vaginal estrogen, frequently helps with bladder problems and vaginal dryness.

Myth #3: Your symptoms will be awful

The fact is that while menopause may not be a fun ride, it also isn't a guarantee that hot flashes will ensue. Menopause symptoms affect about 85% of women, but they differ significantly in frequency and severity, and some go gone in five or even fewer years. For instance, some women experience night sweats, which causes them to wake up and remain awake. Some people sleep through the night by covering themselves with a fan, and they seem to be all right. Women are encouraged to inform their healthcare providers about any bothersome menopause symptoms, such as bladder issues and vaginal dryness that can cause painful sex, as many medications, therapies, and simple lifestyle changes can significantly reduce symptoms. Only about 20% of women will experience hot flashes and night sweats that are so severe that they require prescription medication. "Those are not things that women have to put up with.

Myth #4: Your sexual life is dunzo

The truth is that although symptoms like dryness and low libido can interfere with a woman's sexual life, it doesn't necessarily indicate it's over. Many symptoms that make sex less joyful can be managed, even though almost half of women claim menopause has affected their sex lives. 43% of women say they're having the same amount of sex as usual, and 50% say sex is never uncomfortable. In addition to vaginal dilators, vaginal estrogen, and HRT, a good lubricant can assist in relieving painful penetration, dry vagina, and bladder problems. She advises giving your vagina a voice if you feel that having sex will help you maintain a positive and healthy relationship with yourself or a partner throughout the perimenopause and menopause.

Myth #5: Natural cures work precisely as well as pharmaceutical ones

The fact is that they're not. Many natural therapies for difficult menopausal symptoms have conflicting findings, and some supplements, like kava and evening primrose oil, can be pretty harmful. Some, nevertheless, might be advantageous or, at the very least, safe. For instance, there's proof that melatonin supplements can help with specific sleep issues. The North American Menopause Society notes that black cohosh herb has an excellent safety record and has been proven to aid with hot flashes. However, it shouldn't be taken by those who have liver problems. However, because American supplements are not well-regulated, it is best to avoid trying out a lot of over-the-counter remedies. Please discuss if you could benefit from any of these with your doctor.

Chapter 6

Dear progesterone, I'm sorry I took you for granted

Your body produces fewer reproductive hormones during menopause, which causes your periods to end progressively. Although many people find that their periods have stopped, there might be complex side effects to deal with. Menopause symptoms include hot flashes, vaginal dryness, sleeplessness, and weight gain, to name a few.

These are mild symptoms for some people. Others find them to be so disturbing that they require medical attention. Specific symptoms can be relieved by progesterone, either on its own or in combination with estrogen.

Here are some things to know about the advantages and disadvantages of progesterone or hormone therapy if you're thinking about using them to treat menopause symptoms.

What is progesterone?

One common term for progesterone is the pregnancy hormone. Throughout the reproductive years, progesterone affects how the uterus gets ready for a potential pregnancy. It also affects the supply of breast milk and the development of a mucous barrier surrounding the cervix.

Since progesterone is also involved in many other bodily processes, a decrease in ovarian production can lead to the following symptoms:

- Headaches from migraines
- mood swings
- alterations to bone density
- irregular bleeding

What is understood about menopause symptoms and progesterone therapy?

Hormone replacement therapy is the best treatment for menopause symptoms. The most popular treatment for those without uteruses is estrogen on its own. Because there is evidence that estrogen alone raises the risk of uterine cancer and other major health issues, if you do have a uterus, a combination of progesterone and estrogen is often advised.

Combining progesterone and estrogen usually involves taking pills. Progesterone on its own is also available as a pill that contains progesterone that has been micronized and is quickly absorbed by the body.

Why progesterone and estrogen combined?

Every month, the endometrium, the lining of your uterus, sheds while you are still experiencing menstruation. The endometrium doesn't disappear when your periods cease.

The lining thickens as a result of estrogen use, and endometrial thickness raises the risk of endometrial cancer. According to research, progesterone supplementation lowers the risk of cancer by maintaining the uterine lining's thinness.

Hot flashes are decreased with progesterone.

Progesterone's impact on hot flashes and nocturnal sweats in menopausal women was assessed in 2012.

After monitoring the frequency and intensity of these symptoms, they discovered that taking an oral progesterone dose daily reduced the frequency and intensity of hot flashes and night sweats.

Progesterone also helps with menopause-related sleep problems

Sleep disturbances caused by menopause are among the most bothersome symptoms.

Deep sleep was shown to be of higher quality when 300 mg of progesterone was taken daily at bedtime. It also did not lead to any indications of depression or impairing cognitive function during the day.

This research also supported previous studies' findings that progesterone could lessen the intensity of night sweats, which can cause people to wake up from otherwise sound sleep.

Additionally, progesterone may have some advantages for cognition.

Many people report having memory issues and feeling foggy-headed during the menopause. There is some evidence that if hormone replacement therapy is initiated early in the menopause phase, progesterone may guard against cognitive deterioration.

Progesterone was discovered by some researchers to help menopausal women's verbal and visual memory.

The evidence isn't conclusive. For instance, some research revealed that progesterone had no protective effect on cognition at all. Nevertheless, it's crucial to remember that there is no proof progesterone impairs cognitive function.

Does progesterone therapy have any adverse effects?

Sure. You could encounter any of the following adverse effects, or you might have an allergic reaction to progesterone:

- weariness
- migraine
- nausea or discomfort in the abdomen
- either weight gain or fluid retention
- breast sensitivity
- uterine bleeding

Not everyone should take progesterone. Consult your physician about progesterone substitutes if you:

- Are older than sixty
- Have experienced menopause for more than ten years.
- Possess a family or personal history of breast cancer.
- are more susceptible to liver disease, osteoporosis, blood clots, heart attacks, strokes, dementia

What more could be done to lessen menopause symptoms?

There are other solutions available if you want to lessen menopause symptoms without using hormone therapy.

1. Think about natural goods. Alternatives that are natural, such as evening primrose oil or black cohosh, may help lessen hot flashes and night sweats.

2. Work out frequently. Exercise helps you stay in a healthy weight range, enhances your sleep, and lessens the mood swings and worry that come with menopause.
3. Pay attention to what you eat. Steer clear of alcohol, caffeine, and spicy foods, as these can all cause night sweats and hot flashes.
4. Discover healthy coping mechanisms for stress. Stress can affect your mood and sleep quality. Additionally, it may make hot flashes occur more frequently. To keep your stress under control, think about practicing yoga, meditation, tai chi, breathing techniques, or engaging in a favorite pastime.

The bottom line

Progesterone and estrogen are frequently combined to treat menopausal symptoms. When these two hormones work together, they can lessen menopausal symptoms like night sweats and hot flashes.

Progesterone thins the lining of the uterus, which helps stop endometrial cancer from growing. Progesterone, when taken alone or in combination with estrogen, may also enhance sleep and safeguard specific cognitive abilities.

However, not everyone should use progesterone. Consult a medical expert to find out if it's safe for you. You should be well aware of the benefits and drawbacks of utilizing progesterone to treat menopausal symptoms.

There are natural therapies that can help you if the risks are too significant for you.

Chapter 7

Ketogenic Solutions For Menopause

Some find that changing their diet and lifestyle helps to alleviate the menopausal symptoms. However, as of right now, there is no evidence supporting the specific benefits of the ketogenic diet.

When a woman's periods stop, it is known as the menopause. Perimenopause, which precedes this, is when people are most likely to have symptoms, including hot flashes and night sweats. This is brought on by the body's declining progesterone and estrogen levels. While there is no diet that can prevent a decrease in hormone levels, dietary adjustments can help control the symptoms that may arise from this change. Whether the ketogenic diet can help with this is unknown.

In this chapter will look at the risks and adverse effects of the ketogenic diet and whether it's a good option for women going through menopause. We will also look at different diets that might be beneficial.

A ketogenic or "keto" diet causes the body to enter a state of ketosis. This suggests that the body uses fat as fuel by converting it into ketones. Then, instead of using sugar, these ketones are utilized.

To go into ketosis, a person must drastically reduce their intake of carbs and replace them with fat. The ketogenic diet typically includes:

- 65%–60% fat
- 35–35 percent protein
- 10% to 15% carbohydrates

It's possible for someone on a diet to vary what they consume. They can consume a lot of fruits, vegetables, and healthy fats when they are in ketosis, but they can also consume a lot of red meat and saturated fat.

Is the keto diet good for menopause symptoms?

The keto diet may help in reaching a healthy weight, but it's unclear how it may impact other menopause symptoms.

Impacts on weight gain

Some menopausal women may gain weight due to a reduced metabolism and fluctuating hormone levels.

There is insufficient research on the keto diet's ability to assist women in maintaining a healthy weight throughout menopause. Yet a substantial 2017 research of around 89,000 women ranging in age from 49 to 81, compared the effectiveness of four different diets. Researchers put to the test:

- A diet low in fat
- A diet low in carbohydrates
- A diet based on the Mediterranean
- A diet that complies with the Dietary Guidelines for Americans published by the US Department of Agriculture

Researchers discovered that compared to other diet patterns, those who followed a low-carb diet had a decreased risk of postmenopausal weight gain.

The low-carb diet in this trial, however, restricted daily carbohydrate intake to 163 grams (g). This is far less permissive than the keto diet, which caps carbs at less than 50 g.

Impact on Cravings

During the perimenopause and menopause, people may feel more hungry or have food cravings. The ketogenic diet may help with these symptoms by reducing hunger, according to some studies.

For instance, a 2019 research featuring 40 male and 55 female obese participants, the study examined hunger changes brought on by the ketogenic diet.

Researchers discovered that after eight weeks of the ketogenic diet, the female subjects' levels of the hormone glucagon-like peptide 1, which controls hunger, rose. It's interesting to note that the male participants' levels of this hormone dropped.

However, the study didn't particularly examine how menopause affects appetite suppression. The participants included a mix of pre- and postmenopausal females, with ages ranging from 18 to 65.

Impact on insulin

Insulin sensitivity may drop during menopause. The hormone insulin is in charge of transferring blood sugar into cells. A person at risk for type 2 diabetes may experience elevated blood sugar due to insufficient insulin production.

Insulin levels may be balanced using the ketogenic diet. Studies suggests that eating less carbohydrates can improve insulin sensitivity and result in a decrease in the need for insulin.

In a 2018 study, women with ovarian and endometrial cancer who adopted a 12-week ketogenic diet showed improvements in their insulin sensitivity.

Is keto beneficial for hormone balance?

The effects of the ketogenic diet on diminishing levels of progesterone and estrogen are unknown, as there is currently no research on whether the diet supports or hinders the balance of reproductive hormones after menopause.

Can keto bring you out of menopause?

No, menopause cannot be stopped or reversed by a diet, supplement, or prescription. It is a normal stage of life where the body produces less progesterone and estrogen. Hormone replacement treatment, on the other hand, can restore lost hormones and reduce symptoms.

Keto side effects

There may be adverse effects from the keto diet, particularly in the beginning. The term "keto flu" refers to a group of symptoms that many people get when their bodies go into ketosis. These may consist of:

- headache
- irritability
- weakness
- dehydration
- dizziness
- muscular soreness

It may also be more challenging to get enough of some nutrients when on a ketogenic diet. For instance, one research discovered that people on a ketogenic diet eat less fiber. In an effort to avoid carbohydrates, people may consume fewer fruits and vegetables, which results in a decrease in their intake of vitamins, minerals, and prebiotics. Prebiotic fiber provides sustenance for the gut's good bacteria.

Focusing on sticking to the keto diet and consuming lots of fresh fruit will help to counteract this.

Potential risks of the keto diet

Although studies on the keto diet's long-term effects are still being conducted, some hazards appear to be involved.

1. Kidney stones

Kidney stones may become more common in people following the ketogenic diet. A review and meta-analysis for 2021 concluded that youngsters following a ketogenic diet have a 5.8% chance of developing kidney stones. It is 7.9% in adults.

2. Cardiovascular health

According to specific research, the ketogenic diet raises "bad" cholesterol, often known as low-density lipoprotein or LDL cholesterol. For instance, a single brief research discovered that after three weeks on the ketogenic diet, LDL cholesterol rose by 39%. Furthermore, the LDL cholesterol levels of 59% of research participants were higher than the threshold suggested to prevent cardiovascular disease.

Menopause in and of itself increases the risk of heart disease, so consuming a ketogenic diet during menopause may increase that risk.

3. Bone health

Bone health is also impacted by menopause. Osteoporosis risk rises as a result of decreased bone mineral density brought on by estrogen reduction.

A 2020 study examining the effects of a brief ketogenic diet similarly connected bone density reduction with ketosis. Following the diet for 3.5 weeks, the study monitored 30 athletes and discovered that they were breaking down their bones more than growing new ones.

The subjects' capacity to produce new, healthy bone did not return to normal, the researchers added, even when they resumed their regular diets. There were just five females in this study, and the majority of the participants were men. The participants' average age was 28. To fully understand the potential effects of the keto diet on menopausal women, more research is required.

Other diets for menopause

While many people find that the keto diet requires significant changes in their lifestyle, there are alternative ways to achieve and maintain a healthy weight.

- The Mediterranean diet

The main components of the Mediterranean diet include fruits, vegetables, nuts, and other healthy fats like olive oil. It restricts alcohol, red meat, and saturated fats.

The 2017, Researchers who compared the Mediterranean diet to three other diet types in postmenopausal women discovered that while it was less successful than a low-carb diet, it was still more successful than a low-fat diet in terms of weight loss.

Additionally, a 2021 study discovered that postmenopausal women who followed a Mediterranean diet had increased muscle mass and bone density.

- Plant-based diet

A plant-based diet emphasizes meals generated from plants and steers clear of foods originating from animals. A 2018 study when perimenopausal and menopausal vegans, vegetarians, and omnivores were compared, it was shown that eating a diet high in vegetables and low in meat was associated with fewer uncomfortable menopausal symptoms.

Results from a 2012 study including more than 17,000 menopausal women were comparable. Forty percent of the individuals were asked to follow a low-fat diet that included more whole grains, fruits, and vegetables. These people had three times the likelihood of losing weight and getting rid of menopausal symptoms like night sweats and hot flashes.

High-fat, somewhat protein-rich, and low-carb foods are the mainstays of a ketogenic diet. It puts the body into a metabolic state called ketosis, which promotes weight loss.

Weight gain is one of the menopause symptoms that the keto diet may help with. A ketogenic diet, however, also raises LDL cholesterol, which could be dangerous given that menopause also raises the risk of heart disease. Menopause cannot be reversed; a ketogenic diet can only lessen its effects.

Diets centered around plant-based foods, like the Mediterranean diet, may also be beneficial to women undergoing menopause. Before beginning a new diet, people should see a doctor.

Chapter 8
Meet Your Estrobolome

The Estrobolome: Why is gut health during menopause so crucial?

You hear a lot about gut health, microbiome support, and healthy bacteria, and you assume that in order to support your gut system, you should eat better meals and incorporate more foods that are friendly to the gut. However, are you really aware of why this is so crucial for menopause in particular, let alone for general health?

Over the past ten years, there has been a significant increase in our understanding of how the gut microbiome affects our immune, metabolic, and nervous system functions. Fortunately, for those of us going through menopause, some of this understanding has also helped to clarify some of the symptoms we encounter during the hormonal shift.

The reduction in estrogen levels has an effect on the health of our guts in women going through menopause.

Our digestive tracts harbor a vast ecosystem known as the gut microbiome, which is home to TRILLIONS of microorganisms. The gut microbiome is one of the largest organs in the body, second only to the skin, and it is as individual as a fingerprint.

It's even more potent because the amount of bacteria in it exceeds the number of cells in each of our bodies! The majority of these microorganisms are found in the digestive system and support:

- Break down food
- Protect against pathogens
- Breakdown toxins
- Make vitamins
- Supply the gut with energy

We're all familiar with gut instinct, butterflies in the stomach, and how fear makes our stomachs turn into liquids, but there's now growing evidence that diseases like depression, anxiety, and general mental health are influenced by gut flora. Although the reason for the gut-brain axis has long been unclear, we assumed it existed. But since there is a strong link between your gut and brain—the reason being that we have a "gut feeling" and refer to the gut as our "second brain"—many of the menopausal symptoms you may be experiencing, like mood swings, depression, anxiety, and brain fog, may be related to the state of your gut microbiome.

Our estrogen synthesis and the health of our female reproductive system are influenced by over 60 distinct organisms. We refer to this collection of bacteria and fungus as the estrobolome! Yes, I am aware! Just when we were beginning to understand the concept of "gut microbiome," researchers discovered the astrobleme, which is gradually turning into the Holy Grail of methods to help women cope with menopause more easily.

Thus, think of the effects on our energy, sleep patterns, emotions, hot flashes, and brain function if we concentrate on enhancing our intestinal health! The primary hormone produced by females, estrogen, is regulated by this vast community of bacteria and decreases sharply during menopause. This has a broad effect on our health, contributing to the symptoms mentioned above, along with a host of other problems that cause menopause misery for a significant number of women.

What, then, is an estrobolome exactly?

The gut microbiome contains a biome called the astrobleme that controls how our bodies metabolize estrogen. In order for estrogens to enter the bloodstream and reach other bodily tissues, they must first be converted into their active forms by estrogen-metabolizing enzymes known as beta-glucuronidases. The astrobleme produces precisely the correct quantity of beta-glucuronidase to maintain the balance of estrogen when the gut microbiome is in good health.

But in cases of gut dysbiosis, or bacterial imbalances, the amount of beta-glucuronidase in the body can rise. This means that less estrogen is eliminated from the body, leaving more behind to be recirculated, bind to receptors, and affect different physiological processes—basically reversing the body's natural detoxification process. Oestrogen is essential to numerous bodily functions. It controls the build-up of body fat, energy equilibrium, the ability of females to reproduce, cardiovascular health, bone turnover, and cell division. Gut dysbiosis can affect these processes, change the astrobleme, and interfere with estrogen homeostasis. If we're not careful, this can result in inflammation and eventually more severe chronic disorders. Positively, even though our hormones are out of control, we can still manage to strengthen our digestive system! Modest dietary, lifestyle, and exercise regimen adjustments can have a significant positive impact on gut health. Naturally, maintaining a diverse and healthful diet is crucial, but it might not be sufficient to maintain the estrobolome's diversity. This explains why probiotics may be pretty helpful.

Probiotics are a common sight on grocery store aisles. But what are they precisely, and are they effective?

Live organisms are known as probiotics, and the most popular ones include strains of Lactobacillus and Bifidobacterium. The theory is that these will enter your stomach and settle down in your intestines once you've swallowed them. It has been demonstrated that some strains can effectively prevent depression, slow the loss of bone mass, and lower the risk of developing insulin resistance and diabetes. Numerous other menopause-related issues, including weight control, can be assisted by others.

However, any probiotic won't work. It is crucial that you choose a product that is specially designed to meet the demands of women going through menopause ultimately. Many women also prefer that the high-quality, naturally sourced ingredients in their supplements come from ethical sources.

Chapter 9

Is Detox More Important Than Lifestyle?

In the past, individuals would "detox" or "purify" their bodies by using bloodletting, saunas, leaches, and fasts. There are many purported detox and cleanse programs out there, but because we can't cover them all, we'll stick to detox and cleansing diets.

Usually, one or more of the following are involved:

- A length of time during which one fast (drinking just water, fruit juices, or tea without milk)
- consuming solely liquids
- following a restricted diet, such as consuming only smoothies or specific fruits or vegetables
- using pricey "special" detox powders, shakes, beverages, pills, or herbal remedies
- Enemas, laxatives, and fitness regimens.

Medically speaking, detoxes are ineffective unless they are being performed under medical supervision to treat a life-threatening drug or alcohol addiction. They don't cleanse or detoxify any area of your body, and there isn't any reliable evidence that detoxes are better for medical ailments.

Detox advocates frequently claim that the pain and weakness you may feel during detoxification are caused by "toxins leaving your body," but in reality, you're probably just dehydrated, electrolyte deficient, or not getting enough calories or minerals.

Not only are rigid detoxes monotonous, but they can also be dangerous if they deprive you of vital minerals for an extended period of time.

Those with pre-existing medical issues, especially those with diabetes, may also be at risk when following a detox diet.

Special (medical) diets

You might need to follow a specific diet to assist in managing a medical condition like diabetes or epilepsy. If you have diabetes, you may need to inject insulin to regulate your blood glucose levels or constantly manage your carbohydrate intake.

A ketogenic diet can help people with epilepsy limit their carbohydrate intake and induce ketosis in their bodies. At this point, fat is changed from glucose to ketones and consumed as fuel. For specific individuals, ketosis might lessen the symptoms of epilepsy, including seizures. Consult your doctor before you make any dietary adjustments if you follow a medical diet.

Positives of detox diets

A few parts of detox diets, albeit generally ridiculous, can be good for our health if incorporated into regular eating habits. This entails cutting back on alcohol, sugar, and salt, as well as minimizing the frequency of overindulgence.

Reducing sugar intake

Specific detox diets reduce added or processed sugars. You can obtain enough carbohydrates without adding sugar if you consume enough grains, fruits, and veggies.

According to recommendations from the World Health Organization (WHO), adults should consume no more than 10 percent of their daily energy from sugar or less than 12 teaspoons (50 grams) each day. This covers added sugar, juice, and honey sugars.

Reducing salt intake

Specific detox diets eliminate or severely limit salt or salt supplements. This includes the salt used during the manufacturing or cooking process as well as the salt you add.

The human body needs a small amount of salt, but ingesting too much of it can raise blood pressure. Heart failure, heart attacks, kidney issues, fluid retention, stroke, and osteoporosis are all associated with high blood pressure.

Reducing alcohol intake

Alcohol consumption reduction or cessation is advised by many detox regimens, and this can have positive effects on health. See the Australian guidelines for lowering alcohol-related health hazards.

Loss of weight

If the detox diet is low in calories, you might lose weight, which is good for your health if you're overweight. However, according to specialists, doing so reduces your basal metabolic rate, increasing the likelihood that the weight will return when you resume your regular eating habits.

You own incredible, accessible, integrated detox systems.

Your skin, lungs, liver, and kidneys work nonstop to eliminate anything toxic, hazardous, or undesirable from your body.

The liver is the body's primary filter, cleansing your blood by breaking down poisons into waste products. These waste materials and extra fluid are eliminated from the body via the kidneys.

Sweat is the skin's way of getting rid of extra salts, waste materials, and urea, a byproduct of protein breakdown. The lungs release water vapor, carbon dioxide, and trace amounts of other waste gases.

Being healthy does not need you to "detox." By leading a healthy lifestyle and supporting your body's natural detoxification processes with a diet high in fruits, vegetables, and lean meats and low in processed and sugary foods, you can reap the benefits of detoxification without the adverse effects. You can also avoid alcohol addiction and exercise.

Chapter 10
Move From Surviving To Thriving.

Managing the Menopausal Lifequake

Although it could be easy to put your head down and keep doing what you've always done, doing so frequently results in irritation and a more profound sense of unhappiness. There's a better, more compassionate way.

Admit that it's challenging. Self-compassion is "one of the most effective weapons we have,". That does not, however, imply giving up. It simply entails being kind to yourself as you recover. It's admitting that this is not easy. It's expressing to yourself that "this is kicking my ass" and showing a little self-compassion. The brain experiences a change in neurotransmitters at that precise instant. The stress hormone cortisol is lowered by self-compassion, and as cortisol is down, the neurochemicals that will enable us to handle this problem rise.

Create a system for managing the menopause. Like any other disruptive event in life, the menopausal lifequake can be managed with the aid of a toolkit. Menopause can induce a wide range of symptoms, making management seem overwhelming. Thus, address each symptom separately. Strength training can help if you're losing strength and muscle. Look into treatment options like hormone therapy if hot flashes are interfering with your ability to train and sleep. Taking it one symptom at a time can make you feel more in control and may also help you learn to be gentle with yourself as your body adjusts to its changed surroundings and requires support, understanding, and, oftentimes, patience.

Release the pressure. Sometimes, the best course of action is to remove races or other high-stakes events from the schedule temporarily. That way, you can continue to play the sports you love without having to worry about lines and deadlines. "I usually race a lot, so I took a vacation from it, which removed the pressure, and guess what game I picked up again? The passion for the game.

Look for fresh thrills. You may attend the same strength training class or participate in a specific racing series every time. That's fine as long as it doesn't make you unhappy; you're just doing it because you feel like you "should," and you find yourself negatively comparing your present self to everyone else there or to your past self. That's the moment to look out for anything fresh. Thus, triathletes should consider trying gravel racing. Try your hand at CrossFit if you enjoy strength training. Plan a trek in a stunning, unexplored location.

"A new aim is necessary when you find yourself lacking motivation, feeling disoriented, not reaching your objectives, or not receiving the same results," says Rowan, referring to the complaints of many women going through menopause. Step back and survey your surroundings. What catches your attention? What have you always considered attempting? Look for something that sparks your interest. "Say yes and work it out if something gives you tingles within."

Recall who and what brought you this far. You are still the person who accomplished all of those accomplishments, regardless of the sports or activities you participate in today (or do not). "The qualities that have shaped you into the athlete you are have not changed. Whether you are competing, winning a medal, or even just enjoying your sport, you will always be that athlete. You still possess the fortitude, diligence, and perspective that brought you this far, and it is those qualities that will see you through.

Chapter 11

Effortless Sleep

A Natural Method for Improving Sleep During Menopause.

Though it may not always be simple, keep in mind that these changes in hormones are regular and shouldn't be "fixed" or replaced with hormone replacement treatment (HRT). Having said that, we shouldn't think that managing our unpredictable hormones is a standard or appropriate way to live on our own. Herbs, vitamins, and lifestyle changes are mild ways we may support your body and symptoms during this shift. If we start to pay attention and support our environment, we can really make a difference in one area of our lives: sleep.

Menopause Lifestyle Support for Improved Sleep.

You already know that I adore herbs, but when it comes to getting the sleep you so richly deserve, lifestyle approaches for sleep really shine. In truth, sometimes all you really need is a determination to optimize your lifestyle and make sleep a priority. Here are a few things to mainly focus on when it comes to menopause-related sleep issues; however, there are many more that I address in *Hormone Intelligence.*

Introduce a Wind-Down in the Evening.

Perhaps you were always the kind of person who could get up and go, but as soon as your head hit the pillow, you would fall asleep. Even before perimenopause, it isn't the case for the majority of us. However, this is the perfect moment if you haven't had to incorporate a wind-down ritual into your nightly schedule!

The hours leading up to bed are when good sleep really begins. You really need to make it a daily habit in your lifestyle, not just something you do on occasion. Small actions such as lowering the lights, scheduling self-care activities such as a relaxing bath, keeping a sleep journal to record your worries, and putting down electronics at least an hour before bed (really!) can have a significant impact.

Don't Drink Alcohol (For Real!).

I am aware that perimenopause occasionally entails consuming more red wine on one's own, but there is no escaping the fact that alcohol can seriously impair sleep. The leading cause of hot flashes that I can think of is probably caffeine, which can lower melatonin production by around 20%, even at mild doses up to an hour before bed. Not to mention that it increases your chance of breast cancer and can make you feel melancholy. One of the easiest and fastest ways to get to sleep is to kiss your nightly glass goodbye. All it takes is getting past the psychological barrier of having to let go.

Insider tip: vodka is a cleaner option that is far more accepted than other alcohol, even if it still causes some symptoms in many women. Red wine, including your organic, sulfate-free California Pinot Noir, is the worst offender. Limit it to one drink and avoid plain or added sugar. You can cheat by dividing an ounce between two cups.

Strategize Ahead If You Sweat It Out.

For most of us, the optimal sleeping temperature is 67 degrees Fahrenheit, so try to keep your bedroom temperature no higher than that at night. Additionally, wear only lightweight cotton pajamas and keep blankets that you can effortlessly put on or off when your body temperature fluctuates throughout the night, from hot flashes to nocturnal sweats. Keep a second nightgown by the bed, or sleep in your undies, and take hot flash-specific herbs and nutrients if you sweat profusely.

Herbs and Supplements to Help with Menopause Sleep.

It has been demonstrated that a number of herbs and supplements can promote restful sleep without the adverse side effects of medications. The following herbs and supplements have been examined explicitly in menopause or for a menopausal-specific application, in addition to those listed here for general sleep support.

Melatonin.

As previously noted, as we age, our melatonin levels gradually decrease; for some women, this decrease is significant enough to cause sleep disturbances. Research has demonstrated that melatonin supplementation improves disturbed sleep and other vasomotor symptoms of menopause, such as hot flashes and night sweats, and may delay endocrine aging, which is linked to hormone shifts, in women between the ages of 40 and 60 who are entering the menopausal transition.

Use it as directed: 0.3–3 mg daily.

Magnesium and Calcium.

Magnesium alone or in conjunction with calcium can help induce relaxation and sleep, enhance the quality of sleep, and lower anxiety. It may also aid in preventing perimenopausal bone loss. If you have trouble sleeping due to muscle cramps or restless legs syndrome, magnesium may also be able to help.

Use it as follows: 800 mg of calcium and 300–600 mg of magnesium supplement.

5. HTP,

Many research studies have demonstrated the positive effects of 5-hydroxytryptophan (5-HTP) on sleep. 5-HTP is a precursor to the neurotransmitter serotonin, which is essential for sleep duration and quality. 5-HTP has been shown to reduce the amount of time it takes to fall asleep as well as—heavens rejoice—the frequency of nighttime awakenings. Elevating serotonin levels, an essential sleep inducer, is possible with 5-HTP.

How to use it: A 300–500 mg dose is the usual range for 5-HTP.

Ashwagandha

The herb ashwagandha has its origins in traditional Ayurvedic medicine. It is used to strengthen and calm the nerves, nurture and clear the mind, and encourage sound and restful sleep. It is especially beneficial if you're feeling "tired and wired," and it can also help if you're experiencing stress and anxiety, including if you're having trouble managing insomnia.

How to use it: Take 40–60 drops of the tincture or 500–2000 mg in capsule form or tea form before bed.

Hops

Hops, a major component of beer, reduces hot flashes and encourages sleep, so if you experience both at the same time, this herb might be the one to try. Prenylflavonoids are a class of non-steroidal phytoestrogens found in hops. In a 12-week randomized, double-blind, placebo-controlled study, 67 women going through menopause received either a placebo or a standardized hops extract at a dose of 100 mcg or 250 mcg. The 100 mcg dosage outperformed the placebo after six weeks. Both hop extract dosages resulted in a quicker decline in menopausal symptoms, particularly in terms of the hot flash score.

How to use it: I use the tincture (alcohol extract), 1-2 mL (approximately 40-80 drops), before bed for night sweats because this plant is too harsh for tea. As it may induce sleep, could you not use it right before driving? Hops is not advised if you have risk factors for estrogen receptor-positive breast cancer because of its somewhat estrogenic effects.

Lemon balm, passionflower, and Valerian.

Herbalists have long employed Valerian to promote sleep, but it works best for women who have perimenopausal insomnia. After four weeks of treatment, users report more noticeable increases in their quality of sleep. When taken with passionflower and hops, two additional traditional sleep herbs, or with lemon balm, another herb for anxiety and sleep, its advantages might be even higher. In comparison to a placebo group, Valerian and lemon balm combined resulted in statistically significant improvements in the quality of sleep for 100 women in the 50–60 age range.

More potent still, a study examining passionflower's effects in combination with Valerian and hops found that it had results similar to Ambien but without the risks or adverse effects. Passionflower is helpful for anxiety and helps you feel more refreshed when you wake up by promoting and improving the quality of your sleep.

How to take it: 500 mg of pure Valerian twice a day, 80 mg of lemon balm daily, and 320 mg of passionflower daily. Instead, use 40–60 drops of any or all of these tinctures.

Relora.

Relora, a unique blend of Phellodendron and magnolia, two ancient Chinese herbs, lowers cortisol, enhances energy and sleep, and lessens stress and anxiety. Not only can it assist with stress and sleep, but it may also help boost DHEA, which may help with some of the symptoms of vaginal dryness. This is one of the reasons it is beneficial during the perimenopausal years. When I work with women who are having trouble with their sleep, mood, sense of well-being, or perimenopausal symptoms, I frequently use this combo.

Usage: Take 500 mg before bed.

Try My Herbal BedtimeMix Now!

To help you relax, have this delicious tea one hour before going to bed. Combine one teaspoon of each of the following dried herbs: the leaves of lemon balm, lavender flowers, and chamomile flowers. Steep, covered, for 10 minutes in 1 cup of hot water; sieve and adjust sweetness to taste. Alternatively, try this in place of tea, which can exacerbate the problem if you get up in the middle of the night to urinate. Within an ounce. ½ ounce glass bottle mix. Every one of the subsequent tinctures:

- Passionflower tincture
- Skullcap tincture
- Motherwort tincture
- Lavender tincture

Take half a teaspoon every half an hour for two hours before night. Repeat one or two doses as needed if you wake up during the night.

A woman's life often undergoes further modifications throughout the menopausal transition years. You might be taking on greater responsibility at work, supporting your children as they enter maturity, taking care of aged parents, and thinking back on your own life experience. When you combine all of this with menopause symptoms, you can find it difficult to fall asleep at night.

Poor sleep can be exacerbated by mood swings, especially despair, and hot flashes, especially night sweats. Handling these problems might also aid in handling the symptoms of insomnia.

Melatonin and other over-the-counter sleep aids are used by some women who have difficulty falling asleep. Some people turn to prescription drugs for sleep aids, which can be beneficial if taken occasionally. But these shouldn't be used for an extended period of time as they aren't a treatment for sleep disorders like insomnia.

Insufficient sleep has an impact on every aspect of life. In addition to making you feel agitated or melancholy, sleep deprivation might make you more prone to falls and accidents. Furthermore, rather than the other way around, research now indicates that hot flashes are triggered by waking from sleep. Creating healthy bedtime routines can improve your quality of sleep.

Getting a good night's sleep during the menopausal transition

- Throughout menopause and beyond, here are some tips to help you sleep better:
- Adhere to a regular sleep routine. Set aside time each day to go to bed and wake up.
- If possible, avoid taking naps in the late afternoon or evening. That might keep you up at night.
- Establish a nightly ritual. Some individuals take a warm bath, read a book, or listen to relaxing music.
- Avoid using your computer, mobile device, or television in the bedroom. You could find it difficult to fall asleep because of the brightness of these devices.
- Make sure your bedroom is as quiet as possible and at a reasonable temperature—neither too hot nor too chilly.

- Daily exercise should be done at regular intervals, but not right before bed.
- Steer clear of heavy meals right before bed.
- Avoid caffeine late in the day, which can be found in a lot of coffees, teas, and chocolate.
- Recall that drinking does not promote sleep. A modest amount makes it more difficult to fall asleep.

See your doctor if you are experiencing difficulty falling asleep. If making these adjustments to your nighttime routine doesn't provide the desired level of relief, consider considering cognitive behavioral therapy for insomnia. It has been demonstrated that using a problem-solving approach to treatment can assist women experiencing menopause symptoms to sleep better. You can receive cognitive behavioral therapy in one-on-one sessions or in a class. Make sure the person supervising your therapy is a qualified specialist with a background in supporting women through menopause. A local therapist can be suggested by your doctor.

Chapter 12
Stay Forever Young

Healthy eating and regular exercise are essential for maintaining a youthful and active lifestyle after menopause.

Nutrition after menopause

Your nutritional needs alter as you get older. You should consume roughly 1,000 mg of calcium per day prior to menopause. You should consume up to 1,200 mg of calcium daily after menopause.

Additionally crucial for the development of bones and the absorption of calcium is vitamin D. Spinal fracture risk can be significantly reduced by vitamin D. However, excessive calcium or vitamin D intake, particularly if you already have renal issues, might result in kidney stones, constipation, or stomach pain.

The importance of exercise after menopause

After menopause, a lot of women gain weight. The reason for this could be a decrease in estrogen levels. Increasing your level of activity can help you prevent this weight gain. Frequent exercise helps control weight, strengthens the heart and bones, and lifts your spirits. Osteoporosis, diabetes, high blood pressure, obesity, heart disease, and other conditions are more common in women who do not engage in physical activity. Women who are sedentary may also experience sadness, weak muscles, poor circulation, sleeplessness, and persistent back pain.

Walking, running, swimming, biking, and dancing are examples of aerobic exercises that can help avoid some of these issues. Additionally, it aids in increasing HDL cholesterol, or "good" cholesterol. Both lightweight training and weight-bearing activities like jogging and walking contribute to increased bone mass. Moderate exercise helps postmenopausal women maintain bone mass in the spine and reduces the risk of fractures.

Moreover, exercise elevates mood. The brain releases endorphins, which are hormones. A happier mood lasts for a few hours. The body uses it to combat stress as well.

Before beginning an exercise program, always see your healthcare practitioner, especially if you have been inactive. The ideal workout regimen for you can be suggested by your healthcare professional.

Sex after menopause

Throughout and after menopause, some women lose interest in having sex. Less interest in sex may be exacerbated by menopausal symptoms, including drier vaginal tissues and decreased estrogen levels. On the other hand, vaginal area secretions and suppleness can be restored with estrogen creams and pills. Additionally, using personal lubricants may increase the enjoyment of sex. During perimenopause, women who still experience irregular periods must continue taking birth control. To find out which kind of birth control would be best for you, speak with your doctor.

Staying healthy after Menopause

You can lead a healthy life after menopause by following these tips. See your healthcare provider for further details.

- See your healthcare professional to go over the pros and cons of hormone replacement treatment if you're considering it.
- Avoid smoking. One of the main risk factors for heart disease is smoking.
- Exercise regularly. It is advantageous to engage in even mild activity, such as walking for thirty minutes three times a week.
- Keep your weight in check with a low-sugar, well-balanced diet.
- Manage hypertension by medication or alterations in lifestyle. This will lessen your chance of developing heart disease.
- Utilize regular exercise or relaxation techniques to lessen stress in your life.

Post-Menopause Guidance: Maintaining the Health and Beauty of Your Changing Skin

Post-Menopause Advice

After 50 and after menopause, resetting your metabolism can be a gradual process that takes persistence and patience. The following actions can help you maintain your metabolism:

- Prioritize eating a diet rich in fruits, vegetables, whole grains, lean protein, and healthy fats.
- Include regular exercise in your regimen, focusing on aerobic and strength training activities to help you gain muscle mass.
- Drink lots of water throughout the day to stay hydrated.
- Make getting enough sleep a priority to help your metabolism and general wellness.
- Reduce stress by practicing yoga, meditation, or other relaxation techniques. Keep in mind that each person's body is different, so for individualized advice, it's crucial to speak with a healthcare provider or nutritionist.

Menopause and Skincare: Use These Tips to Fight Skin Changes

It's like a hot bath in life. The longer you stay in it, the more wrinkled you get, even if it feels amazing while you're in it. Who can understand?

Aging has numerous advantages, like fulfilling work, raising larger families, enjoying a luxurious retirement, spoiling grandkids, and endless wisdom. *frown wink*

But becoming older is not without its difficulties, particularly for women. As we get older, those hormones that once made us miraculous, life-giving goddesses start to rebel against us and pose problems.

Together with some professional advice on how to take care of your skin both during and after menopause, let's examine why and how your skin changes with age.

Why Does My Skin Feel And Look Different During Menopause?

How does menopause affect the skin? Estrogen is the most straightforward answer to this query. The generation of estrogen and progesterone that a woman's body would typically produce in a monthly cycle slows down and finally stops when ovarian production diminishes and becomes erratic in her mid-to late-40s. Menopause is thought to have begun when the periods have stopped for a continuous twelve months. This slowing stage is known as perimenopause or before-menopause.

Regretfully, because of the altered hormone ratios in your body, you can start to experience alterations even during the slow-down phase. Hormonal changes will affect every system in the body, but the skin will typically exhibit the most noticeable effects.

The hydration and retention of skin lipids are primarily dependent on estrogens. This is the reason why you could experience abnormally dry skin. The generation of collagen by the body, which is essential for the strength, firmness, and suppleness of the skin, is also negatively impacted by the decline in estrogen. Together with new or worsened fine lines and wrinkles, sagging skin can also result from a loss of fat beneath the skin's surface.

Maybe by now, you're hoping that Peter Pan will take you to Never-Never Land and grant you eternal youth. You are not to blame. It's not all terrible news, either. For our go-to advice on preserving your naturally gorgeous skin as long as possible, keep reading.

Professional Advice for Your Skin After Menopause

Keeping your skin (and body) feeling its best after menopause can be achieved with these easy tips from our experts. Consume a wide variety of foods, including some essential fats, stay hydrated, move your body, and get plenty of sleep.

The vibrantly colored rainbow of fruits and vegetables seen in nature is rich in antioxidants, which our bodies require to remain healthy from the inside out. We advise consuming a broad range of foods and making an effort to consume every hue in the rainbow! Essential fatty acids are yet another critical element in maintaining your optimal appearance. They function from the inside out to support the maintenance of your skin's oil barrier, which is compromised during menopause. Soy, flax, walnuts, sardines, and salmon are excellent sources of these essential omega-3 fatty acids. Do you feel peckish yet?

Speaking of our body healing itself from the inside out, let's discuss the importance of water. Increasing the amount of water in our bodies should help alleviate dry skin if that is the case. Please fill up your preferred reusable water bottle and carry it with you for convenient access to on-the-go hydration. Your skin and body will appreciate it, we promise.

Our needs—and maybe even desires—for exercise vary as we get older. Even though the majority of us aren't participating in our favorite sports, running marathons, or competing as athletes anymore, we should still be active. One thing that remains constant despite our changing requirements is the body's urge to move.

Exercise improves circulation, which increases the amount of nutrients that reach your skin. This is beneficial for your heart and bones. Additionally, this can boost the creation of collagen and elastin, which is essential for skin suppleness and which, as we previously said, considerably declines due to declining estrogen levels.

Get some sleep now; you deserve it. Sleeping for the recommended seven to nine hours each night lowers stress levels and helps avoid dark bags beneath the eyes. Additionally, it aids in your body's recharging so that you can wake up feeling and looking renewed.

Now that your diet, exercise, and sleep are all at their best, let's go one step further and make sure your beauty routine is excellent as well.

Step-by-Step Guide to Post-Menopause Beauty Regime

You probably know the majority of the components of a good skincare and cosmetic routine by now. During this stage of life, there can be some fresh aspects of your beauty routine that are worth giving another look.

Step 1: Cleanse

Did you know, for instance, that warm water tends to moisturize skin more than hot water? Because of this, reduce the temperature while washing your skin in order to prevent losing essential moisture during this fundamental step of skin care. It's all to support the cause. Therefore, you should also use a mild cleanser that is designed to eliminate impurities without drying out or irritating the skin!

Step 2: Polish

Next, skin discoloration where age spots or uneven skin tones may be present might be helped by mild exfoliation to eliminate excess dead skin cells. Take caution not to overdo this process by exfoliating too much; instead, find out what works best for you by speaking with a dermatologist or healthcare expert.

Step 3: Hydrate and Treat

The next step is to target the fine lines and wrinkles. This can assist the skin in removing damaged collagen and elastin, thereby supporting the skin's natural capacity to repair and renew itself and preserve healthy skin. Treating your skin can help to reduce the appearance of wrinkles, as well as level out skin tone and restore volume to the skin.

You may have noticed a recurring theme of hydration and moisture. The best results will be obtained by applying a moisturizer to specific areas of the face and neck. To achieve the most outstanding results, moisturizing twice daily is recommended. Get an oil-free product that soothes, nourishes, and moisturizes the skin while also addressing the elusive collagen and elastin. Because the skin on the neck and décolleté is more sensitive, they require exceptional support. The same is true for our eyes if you've ever debated whether or not you need a separate eye cream.

Step 4: Safeguard

The final component of your beauty routine is undoubtedly the most significant and long-lasting beauty tip: sunscreen. Whether the sky is dark and overcast or the sun is shining brightly, sunscreen should be worn at all times by people of all ages. Hormonal changes in the skin during menopause can impair your skin's natural sun protection, and we all know that nothing reveals wrinkles and aging like time in the sun.

If you're reading this while relaxing in a warm bath, it's time to get out and moisturize! This has given you some ideas for keeping your skin appearing natural and lovely as you get older.

Conclusion

You can achieve a comprehensive lifestyle reset to decrease disruptive menopause symptoms by following a ketogenic diet, intermittent fasting, focused exercise, restorative sleep, stress management, hormone support, and gut healing. Balance blood sugar, metabolism, hormones, and inflammation in this way to feel steady, energized, and vibrant during the shift. You may regain control of your health via food, lifestyle modifications, mental support, and medical direction and thrive through perimenopause, menopause, and beyond.